ACKNOWLEDGMENTS

First and foremost I'd like to thank Jesus Christ for giving me the vision, energy and patience to start and complete this book.

My five beautiful children, Dominique, Briana, Brittney, Jaeda and Zion for being the main motivating factors for this project. My mother, Doris; my pop, Scottie and Grandma Eula- Mae. Antioch Baptist Church of Jamaica, NY (my church family), Talk of the Town Toastmasters, St. Albans, Queens, the poets in my book, family, friends and anyone who had anything to do with helping bring my dream of becoming an author to fruition.

Grateful acknowledgement and special thanks to Jacqueline Carr - author of **A Selected Few Just For You,** who has worked diligently in formatting and typing the material for this book. Also worth mentioning is St. Albans Printing - Queens, New York, who is responsible for my book design; and lastly special thanks to my friends and print professionals at SavMore Digital Printing - Brooklyn, New York.

DEDICATION

This is dedicated to my grandmother, Mrs. Paralee Scott: who inspired me when she was alive in the physical, and now in the spirit smiled and approved my work from heaven.

In memory of my sister Valerie Monique Blackman

My 100 Favorite Fitness Words

1. **<u>ABDOMEN (ABS)</u>** – Stomach, below the chest that contains other organs including stomach, between the thorax and the pelvis.

2. **<u>Aerobics</u>** – A system of physical conditioning involving exercises (as running, walking, swimming, or calisthenics) performed to temporary increase in respiration and heart rate.

3. **<u>Amino Acids</u>** – Anyone of many acids that occur naturally in living cells which form proteins.

4. **<u>Apparatus</u>** – A piece of equipment used for specific physical activities.

5. **<u>Bands</u>** – A rubber cord that confines or constricts while allowing a degree of movement. Resistance, work-out bands.

6. **<u>Beast Mode</u>**- To get into a zone (Apex) of a particular exercise, to be in a highly motivated mood.

7. **Bench Press** – A lift of exercise in which a weight is raised by extending the arms upward while lying on a bench.

8. **Belt** – Weight lighting belt, worn around the waist to support the back while lifting.

9. **B.M.I** (Body Mass Index) – An index for assessing overweight underweight, obtained by dividing body weight in kilograms by height in meters squared.

10.   **<u>Breathe</u>** – To take air, oxygen, etc., into the lungs and expel inhale and exhale. Normal respiration is important in maintaining good health and wellness.

11.   **<u>Calisthenics</u>**- Gymnastic type exercises designed to develop physical health and vigor. The art and practice of exercises.

12.   **<u>Calories</u>** – A quantity of food capable of producing such and amount of energy.

13.   **<u>Cardio</u>** – A combining form meaning "heart" etc. Cardiogram, Cardiovascular affecting the heart and blood vessels.

14.   **<u>Challenge 30 day</u>**- A commitment to do a certain exercise or exercises for 30 straight calendar days. (30 day AB challenge, 30 day leg challenge, etc.)

15.   **<u>Conditioning</u>** – Enhancement of heart and circulatory function produced by regular aerobic exercise such as jogging, swimming or cycling.

16. **Commitment** – The act of committing, pledging or engaging oneself. Pledge, obligation or discipline. When pertaining to exercise, to reach a goal of weight loss, weight gain, diet, etc.

17. **Carbohydrates** – Organic compounds that change to substances on simple chemical that form supporting tissues of plants and that is important food for people.

18. **Core** – The central, innermost, or most essential part of anything. Pertaining to exercising the body, the abdominal section of one's body is the core.

19. **Consultation** – A meeting with a fitness instructor for discussion or seeking or advice to help with exercise and /or diet goals.

20. **Circuit** – A form of high-intensity aerobics and exercise with machines normally in a timely manner, mostly with 30 – 60 second breaks in between.

21. **<u>Crossfit</u>** – Branded fitness regimen created by Greg Glassman, a physical exercise philosophy, strength and conditioning program.

22. **<u>Crunches</u>** – An abdominal exercise that works the rectus abdominal muscle and also works the obliques.

23. **<u>Diet</u>** – The food intake of an organism, Nutrition, Formal deliberative assembly.

24. **Digestive System** – A multistage process starting from ingestion of raw materials, most often other organisms. Usually involves some type of mechanical and chemical processing. Digestion is separated into four steps.

25. **Dumbbells** – A type of free weight, is a piece of equipment used in with training, used individually or in pairs.

26. **Energy** – Technically it is the "ability of a system to perform the capacity of vigorous activity, an exertion of power.

27. **<u>Endurance</u>** – to exert and remain active for a long period of time strength to continue despite fatigue, stress, etc. Lasting quality.

28. **<u>Electrolytes</u>** – Any substance that dissociates into ions when dissolved in a suitable medium or melted and thus forms a conductor of electricity. Such drink as Gator-Aid, Vitamin water, etc. has Electrolytes.

29.   **<u>Elliptical Machine</u>** – An exercise machine like a stationary bike without a seat, done in an upright position.

30.   **<u>Effort</u>**- The amount of exertion/energy expended for a specific purpose, a strenuous attempt.

31.   **<u>Equilibrium</u>** – A state of rest or balance, mental or emotional Equanimity.

32. **<u>Exercise</u>** – Any bodily activity that enhances or maintains physical fitness and overall health and wellness. Including increasing Growth and development, preventing aging, strengthening muscles and cardiovascular.

33. **<u>Focus</u>** – Selectively concentrating, to give maximum attention & effort.

34. **<u>Free Weights</u>** – Consisting of dumbbells, bar bells and exercise machines, or equipment that is not connected to an Apparatus.

35.   **Gear** –Fitness and exercise clothing from gloves to shirt and pants to sneakers.

36.   **Goals** – An objective that a person plans or intends to achieve.

37.   **Glutes** – Gluteus Maximus known as Glutes. The main extensor muscle of the hip.

38.   **Gym** – Gymnasium, an indoor fitness facility.

39.   **<u>Fit</u>** – Being in good physical condition. In good health.

40.   **<u>Hydration</u>** – The process of providing an adequate amount of water to body tissues.

41.   **<u>Health</u>** – General condition of the body or mind with reference to soundness, vigor and vitality.

42.   **<u>Instructor</u>** – A qualified fitness professional who helps and assist in exercise regimen.

43.   **Jacuzzi** – A hot tub or whirlpool bath with underwater jets that massage the body.

44.   **Jog** – An energetic trot, slower than a run.

45.   **Kettle Bells** – A weight consisting of a cast iron ball with a single handle for gripping the weight during exercise.

46. **Kickboxing (Karate**) - A form of boxing in which competitors use gloves and may also kick with bare feet, a strenuous exercise.

47. **Lifting** – A form of exercise in which weights are lifted.

48. **Leg Lifts** – Exercise legs with gym machines with weights in a sitting position.

49.   **Longevity** – The quality of being long-lasting, especially in life (Exercise can give you that).

50.   **Mass** – Bulk, magnitude, excess body weight, especially in the form of muscle hypertrophy.

51.   **Machines** – A gym device that directs and controls muscle movement and energy to produce a certain effect.

52.   **Mat**- A floor pad to protect exercises while engaging in different forms i.e., yoga, stretching, etc.

53.   **Motivation**- Incentive to do something, to encourage "Go Hard" while lifting weights or exercising.

54.   **Mindfulness** – Awareness, inclination to be mindful. (Imperative to your health and wellness).

55. **Metabolism** – The complete set of chemical reactions that occur in living cells.

56. **Muscle** – A well-development physique, in which the muscles are enlarged from exercise. (An organ composed of muscle tissue).

57. **Nutrition**- The organic process by which an organism assimilates food and uses it for growth and maintenance. Nourishment to give energy and build tissue.

58.   **Partner** – A person associated and assisting another while exercising.

59.   **Physicality** – Having physical attributes especially when overdeveloped, preoccupation with the body and physical needs.

60.   **Pounds (lbs)** - A unit of mass and weight, (How many pounds do you weigh?) Essential to how much weight you can lift and other limits while exercise.

61.   **Protein** – Any of numerous large, complex naturally-produced molecules composed of one more long chains of acid.

62.   **Pilates**- A system of physical conditioning involving low-impact exercises and stretches designed to strengthen muscles of the torso and often performed with specialized equipment.

63.   **Pull-ups**- An exercise consisting of chiming oneself, as on a horizontal bar.

64.   **Push-ups**- An exercise in which a person, keeping a prone position with the hands palms down under the shoulder, normally pushing up your own weight.

65.   **Quads** – Quadriceps muscles, a large muscle in front of the thigh.

66.   **Regimen** – A regulated course as of diet, exercise or manner of living, intended to preserve or restore health or to attain some result.

67.   **Repetition** – The act of repeating an action, doing the same exercise of production and performance.

68.   **Release** – A freeing or releasing from pain, emotional strain or stress. (Exercising is one of the very best stress relievers.)

69.   **Rest** – Refreshing ease or inactivity after extortion or labor, tranquility, solitude.

70.   **Results** – An outcome, something that happens as a result of a certain action. (In the fitness world for exercising.)

71.   **Ripped** – Slang for a "muscled body" from the results of lifting weights or doing Calisthenics.

72.   **Rowing** – (Machine) – An exercise machine having a mechanism with two oars like handles, foot braces, and sliding seat. The motions of rowing.

73.   **<u>Sauna</u>** – A bath that uses dry heat to induce perspiration and in which steam is produced by pouring water on heated stones.

74.   **<u>Sets</u>** – An amount of a certain exercise done in between a break of a set number of said exercise (3 "sets" of 25 push-ups equal 75 pushup.

75.   **<u>Spot</u>**- To have the support of a person while lifting weights on a weight bench.

76.   **<u>Squats</u>** – A weightlifting exercise in which a person squats and then returns to an erect position while holding a barbell at the back of shoulders.

77.   **<u>Steam Room</u>** – A steam filled and heated room to induce sweating, as in a Turkish bath.

78.   **<u>Strength</u>** – The quality or state of being strong, bodily or muscular power, vigor. Having mental and physical power.

79.   **Stretch** – To draw out or extend (oneself, a body, limbs wings, etc.) to the full length or extent.

80.   **Studio** – A room or place for instruction or experimentation for any form of exercise, dance, etc.

81.   **Supplements** – Something added to complete a thing, supply a deficiency, or reinforce or extend a whole. (Relating to diet, vitamins in a fitness, health & wellness.)

82. **<u>Swimming</u>** – To move in water by movements of the limbs, to float on the surface of water. (Great for cardio, lungs and overall body workout.)

83. **<u>Sweat (Perspiration)</u>** – To perspire freely, to exude moisture from the body.

84. **<u>Taebo</u>** – Created by Billy Blanks, in the 1990's. A totally body fitness that incorporates martial arts techniques, TAE (Taekwondo) BO (Boxing) A cardio boxing program.

85.   **Testosterone** – Secreted by the testes, that stimulates the development of male organs.

86.   **Massage** – Working acting on the body with pressure, used to promote relaxation and well-being and is beneficial in treating injuries or other problems affecting the masculative of body.

87.   **Trainer** – A person who trains athletes, and gym members, one who also is qualified to give advice on exercising; and who gives first aid and therapy.

88.   **Treadmill** – An exercise machine that allows the user to walk or run in place, usually on a continuous moving belt.

89.   **Triceps** – A muscle having three heads or points of origin, especially the muscle on the back of the arm.

90.   **Tone (Body Tone)** - To gain or cause to gain in tone or strength strengthening or tightening up the body or certain muscle.

91.   **<u>Vitamins B (Energy)</u>** – Any of a group of organic substances essential in small qualities to normal metabolism, found in food or produced synthetically.

92.   **<u>Water</u>** – A transparent, odorless, tasteless liquid, a compound of hydrogen and oxygen (H_2O). (The very best and healthiest liquid for the body.)

93.   **<u>Walking</u>** – To move about or travel on foot for exercise, pleasure or travel (The most common form of exercise assisting in losing weight. Other benefits.)

94.   **<u>Weight loss</u>** – Dropping down in pounds from one's body weight.

95.   **<u>Wellness</u>** – The quality or state of being healthy in body and mind. An approach to healthcare that emphasizes preventing illness and prolonging life.

96.   **<u>Yoga</u>** – A series of postures and breathing exercises practiced to achieve control of the body and mind, tranquility, etc.

97. **<u>Zone</u>** – A state of intense concentration and focus that greatly improves a person's performance in a physical or mental activity.

98. **<u>Zumba</u>** – A brand name for a fitness program consisting of dance and aerobic exercise routines performed to popular, mainly Latin-American music.

99.   **Referee** (Basketball) – Believed to be the most productive workout for stamina in all of officiating sporting events, running up and down a basketball court for a minimum of an hour (constant running or walking.)

100. **Membership** – To belong to a fitness facility, access to a gym normally for a fee.

"Exercise has physical, mental, emotional, spiritual and financial benefits. If you want to naturally look good, feel good and have confidence everyday just exercise regularly".

EZ Blackman

DELICIOUS SMOOTHIES

SERVINGS: 1

1½ c chopped strawberries

1 c blueberries

½ c raspberries

2 Tbsp honey

1 tsp fresh lemon juice

½ c ice cubes

BLEND all ingredients.

NUTRITION (*per serving*) *162.5 cals, 1 g fat, 0.1 g sat fat, 5 mg sodium, 41.5 g carbs, 32 g sugars, 6 g fiber, 2 g protein*

MORE: 7 Ways To Boost Your Energy Without Caffeine

Sunrise Smoothie

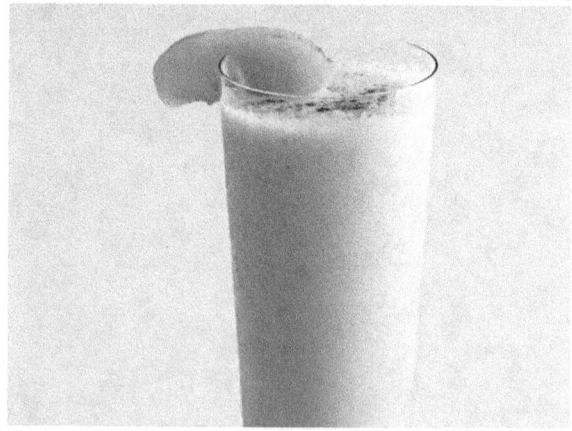

Blend apricot and peach together, and your smoothie will look like an early-morning sunrise.

SERVINGS: 4

1 banana

1 c apricot nectar, chilled

1 container (8 oz) low-fat peach yogurt

1 Tbsp frozen lemonade concentrate

½ c club soda, chilled

1. COMBINE the banana, apricot nectar, yogurt, and lemonade concentrate. Process for 30 seconds, or until smooth and creamy.

2. STIR in the club soda and serve immediately.

NUTRITION (*per serving*) *130 cals, 0.5 g fat, 0.5 g sat fat, 43.5 mg sodium, 29 g carbs, 16 g sugars, 1.5 g fiber, 2.5 g protein*

MORE: This Drink Recipe Lowers Blood Pressure

Berry Vanilla Sensation

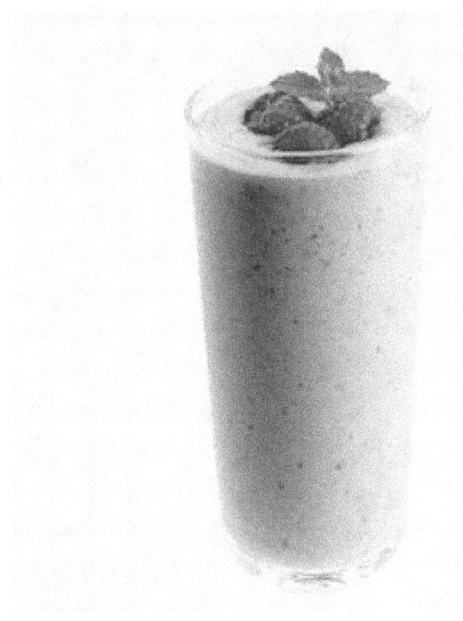

Fat-free vanilla yogurt sweetens this tangy fruit healthy smoothie recipe.

SERVINGS: 2

½ c frozen unsweetened raspberries

½ c frozen unsweetened strawberries

¾ c unsweetened pineapple juice

1 c (8 oz) fat-free vanilla yogurt

COMBINE the raspberries, strawberries, and pineapple juice. Add the yogurt. Blend until smooth.

NUTRITION (*per serving*) *192 cals, 0.5 g fat, 0.1 g sat fat, 86.5 mg sodium, 41 g carbs, 35 g sugars, 2.5 g fiber, 7 g protein*

MORE: 3 Post-Workout Drinks That Help Your Muscles Recover

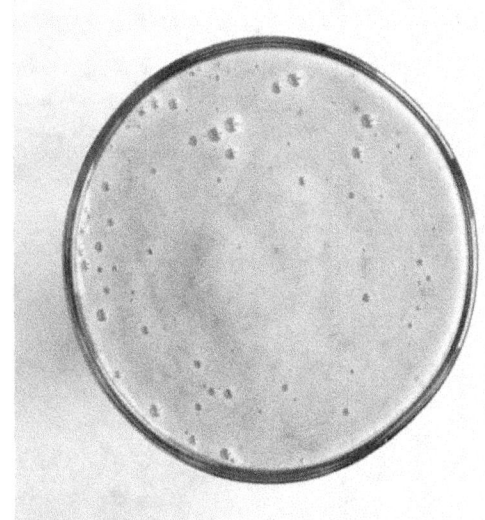

Tutti-Frutti Smoothie

A splash of orange juice infuses summer citrus into this healthy and refreshing snack.

SERVINGS: 2

½ c loose-pack mixed frozen berries or strawberries

½ c canned crushed pineapple in juice

½ c plain yogurt

½ c sliced ripe banana

½ c orange juice

COMBINE the berries, pineapple (with juice), yogurt, banana, and orange juice in a food processor fitted with the metal blade, in a blender, or in a large measuring cup with an immersion blender. Process for about 2 minutes, or until smooth.

NUTRITION (*per serving*) *140 cals, 2.5 g fat, 1.5 g sat fat, 30 mg sodium, 29 g carbs, 16 g sugars, 2.5 g fiber, 3.5 g protein*

MORE: 25 Snacks That Won't Leave You Hungry
LeeAnn's Luscious Smoothie

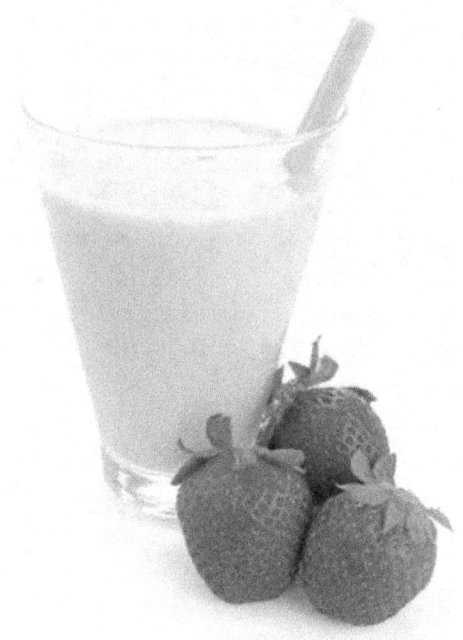

LeeAnn's Luscious Smoothie

To eliminate processed sugar, this reader created a sweet, sugar-free smoothie.

SERVINGS: 1

1 c skim milk

1 c frozen, unsweetened strawberries

1 Tbsp cold-pressed organic flaxseed oil

1 Tbsp sunflower or pumpkin seeds (optional)

1. MIX milk and frozen strawberries in a blender for 1 minute.

2. TRANSFER to a glass and stir in the tablespoon of flaxseed oil, or serve with a tablespoon of sunflower or pumpkin seeds instead.

NUTRITION (*per serving*) *256 cals, 14 g fat, 1.5 g sat fat, 106 mg sodium, 26 g carbs, 19 g sugars, 3 g fiber, 9 g protein*

MORE: This Is Your Body On Sugar (Infographic)

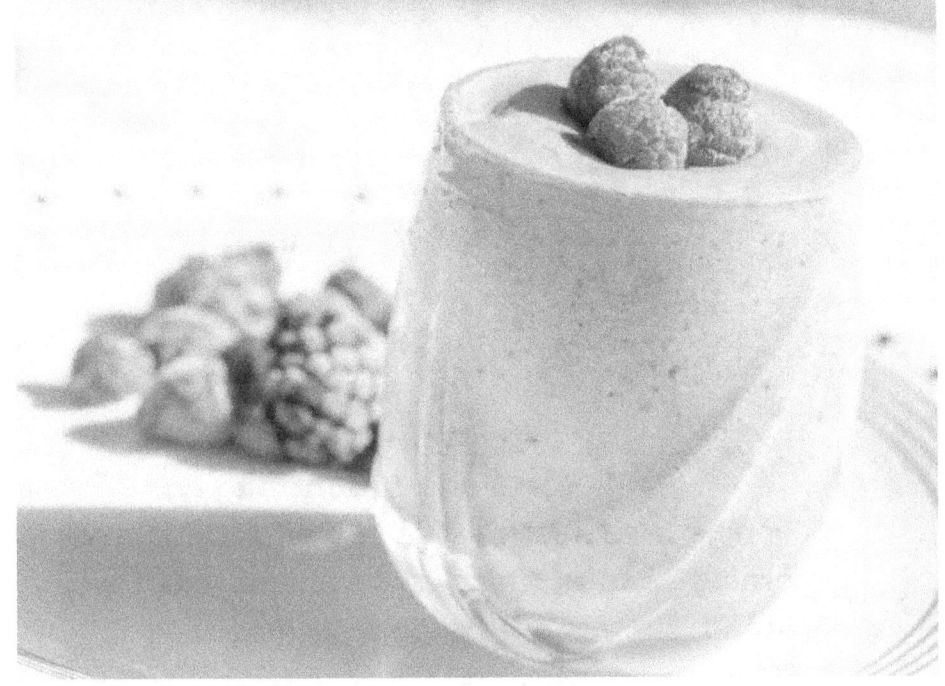

Slim-Down Smoothie

Wonderfully thick and tasty, this healthy smoothie recipe easily substitutes for milkshakes and ice cream.

SERVINGS: 1

1 c frozen berries, such as blueberries, raspberries, or strawberries

½ c low-fat yogurt (any flavor)

½ c orange juice or other juice

PLACE the berries, yogurt, and orange juice in a blender and pulse for 30 seconds. Blend for 30 seconds, or until smooth.

NUTRITION (*per serving*) *185 cals, 2 g fat, 1 g sat fat, 90 mg sodium, 35 g carbs, 26 g sugars, 3.5 g fiber, 8 g protein*
MORE: The 11 Healthiest Drinks Of All Time

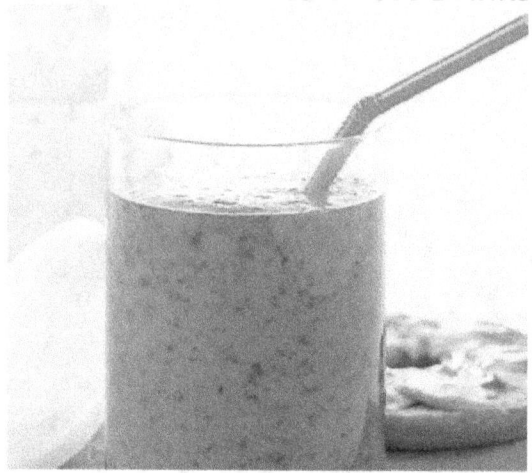

Soy Good Smoothie

Skipping breakfast can leave you starving mid-morning—and reaching for tempting junk food. Instead, sip this on-the-go soy smoothie.

SERVINGS: 1

1 c calcium-fortified vanilla soy milk

½ c frozen blueberries

½ c corn flakes cereal

1 frozen banana, sliced

COMBINE the milk, blueberries, cereal, and banana in a blender for 20 seconds. Scrape down the sides and blend for an additional 15 seconds.

NUTRITION (*per serving*) *350 cals, 3.5 g fat, 0.1 g sat fat, 192 mg sodium, 74 g carbs, 44 g sugars, 7 g fiber, 9 g protein*
MORE: 5 Surprisingly Easy DIY Dairy-Free Milks

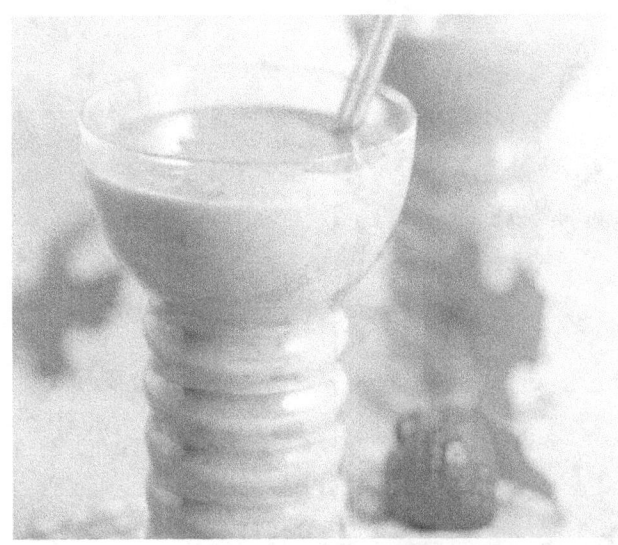

Strawberry-Kiwi Smoothie

Stay full and fight disease. This high-fiber smoothie recipe becomes even healthier when you use organic kiwis, which contain higher levels of heart-healthy polyphenols and vitamin C.

SERVINGS: 4

1¼ c cold apple juice

1 ripe banana, sliced

1 kiwifruit, sliced

5 frozen strawberries

1½ tsp honey

COMBINE the juice, banana, kiwifruit, strawberries, and honey. Blend until smooth.

NUTRITION (*per serving*) *87 cals, 0.3 g fat, 0 g sat fat, 3.5 mg sodium, 22 g carbs, 16.5 g sugars, 1.5 g fiber, 0.5 g protein*

Orange Dream Creamsicle

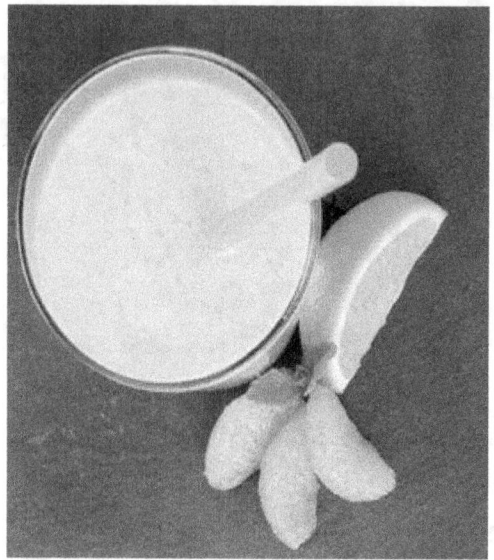

Need to cool down after a tough workout or a hot day at the beach? Lap up this low-cal, citrus-infused drink.

Servings: 1

- 1 navel orange, peeled
- ¼ c fat-free half-and-half or fat-free yogurt
- 2 Tbsp frozen orange juice concentrate
- ¼ tsp vanilla extract
- 4 ice cubes

Combine the orange, half-and-half or yogurt, orange juice concentrate, vanilla, and ice cubes. Process until smooth.

Nutrition *(per serving) 160 cals, 3 g protein, 36 g carbs, 3 g fiber, 28 g sugars, 1 g fat, 0.5 g sat fat, 60 mg sodium*

Tropical Papaya Perfection

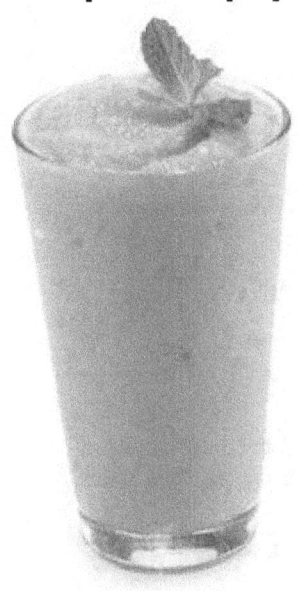

Thick like a milkshake, this coconut-infused smoothie transports you to a tropical island.
Servings: 1

- 1 papaya, cut into chunks
- 1 c fat-free plain yogurt
- ½ c fresh pineapple chunks
- ½ c crushed ice
- 1 tsp coconut extract

- 1 tsp ground flaxseed

Combine the papaya, yogurt, pineapple, ice, coconut extract, and flaxseed. Process for about 30 seconds, or until smooth and frosty.
Nutrition (*per serving*) *299 cals, 1.5 g fat, 0.1 g sat fat, 149 mg sodium, 64 g carbs, 44 g sugars, 7 g fiber, 13 g protein*

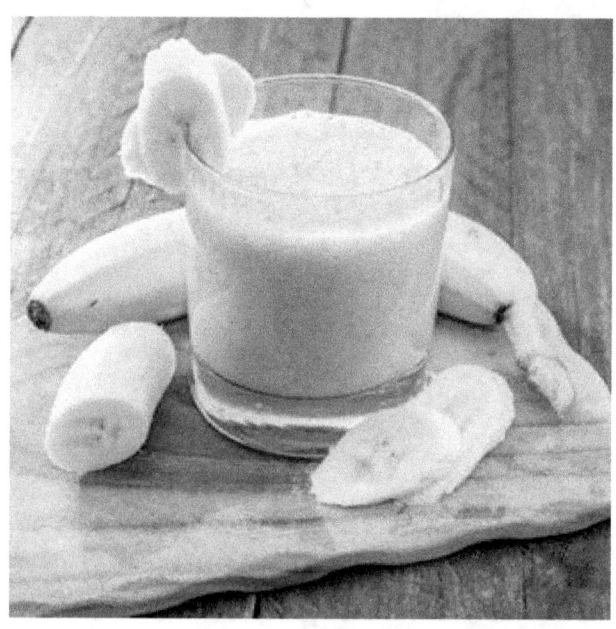

Banana Ginger Smoothie
Soothe digestion, heartburn, nausea, and other stomach trouble with the fresh ginger in this natural remedy drink.
Servings: 2

- 1 banana, sliced
- ¾ c (6 oz) vanilla yogurt
- 1 Tbsp honey
- ½ tsp freshly grated ginger

Combine the banana, yogurt, honey, and ginger. Blend until smooth.

Nutrition (*per serving*) *157 cals, 1 g fat, 0.8 g sat fat, 57 mg sodium, 34 g carbs, 28 g sugars, 1.5 g fiber, 5 g protein.*

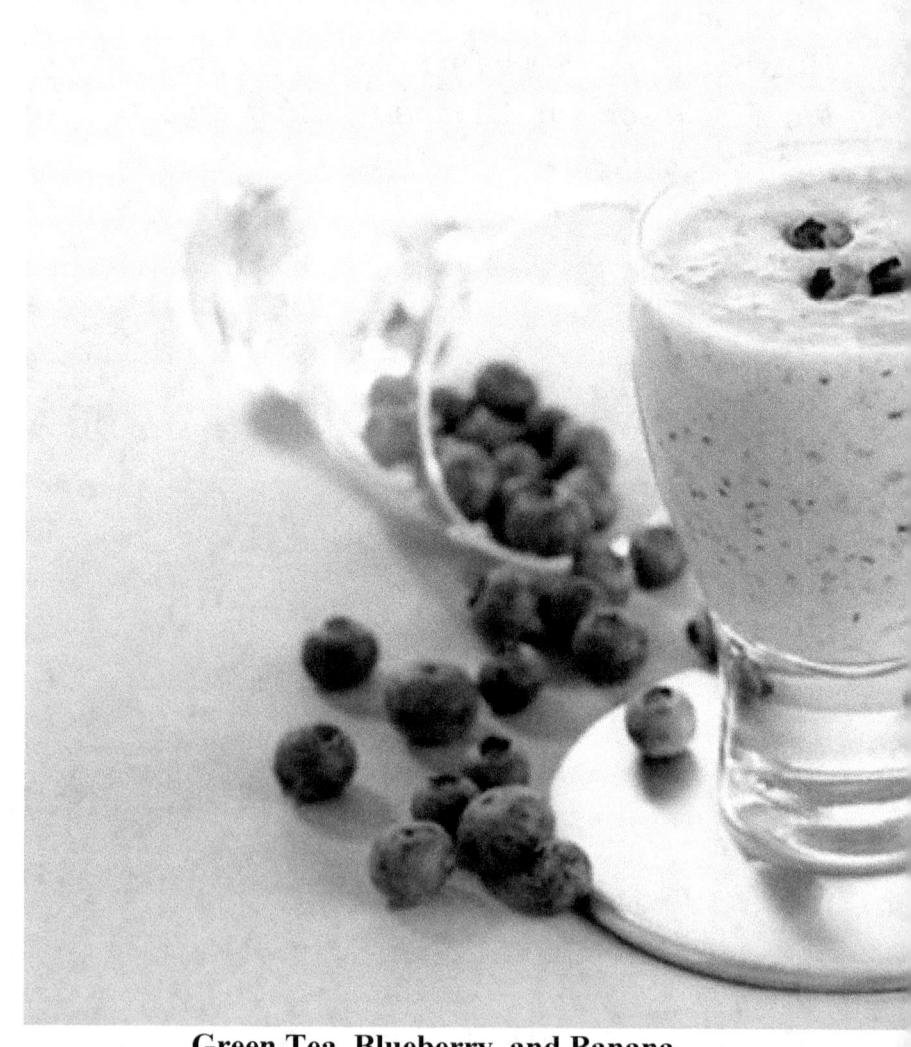

Green Tea, Blueberry, and Banana

Antioxidant-rich green tea makes this healthy smoothie a nutritional powerhouse.

SERVINGS: 1

3 Tbsp water
1 green tea bag
2 tsp honey
1½ c frozen blueberries
½ med banana
¾ c calcium fortified light vanilla soy milk

1. MICROWAVE water on high until steaming hot in a small bowl. Add tea bag and allow to brew 3 minutes. Remove tea bag. Stir honey into tea until it dissolves.
2. COMBINE berries, banana, and milk in a blender with ice crushing ability.
3. ADD tea to blender. Blend ingredients on ice crush or highest setting until smooth. (Some blenders may require additional water to process the mixture.) Pour smoothie into tall glass and serve

NUTRITION (per serving) 269 cals, 2.5 g fat, 0.2 g sat fat, 52 mg sodium, 63 g carbs, 38.5 g sugars, 8 g fiber, 3.5 g protein

MORE: 11 Tasty Ideas With Fresh Blueberries

4/21

Very Berry Breakfast

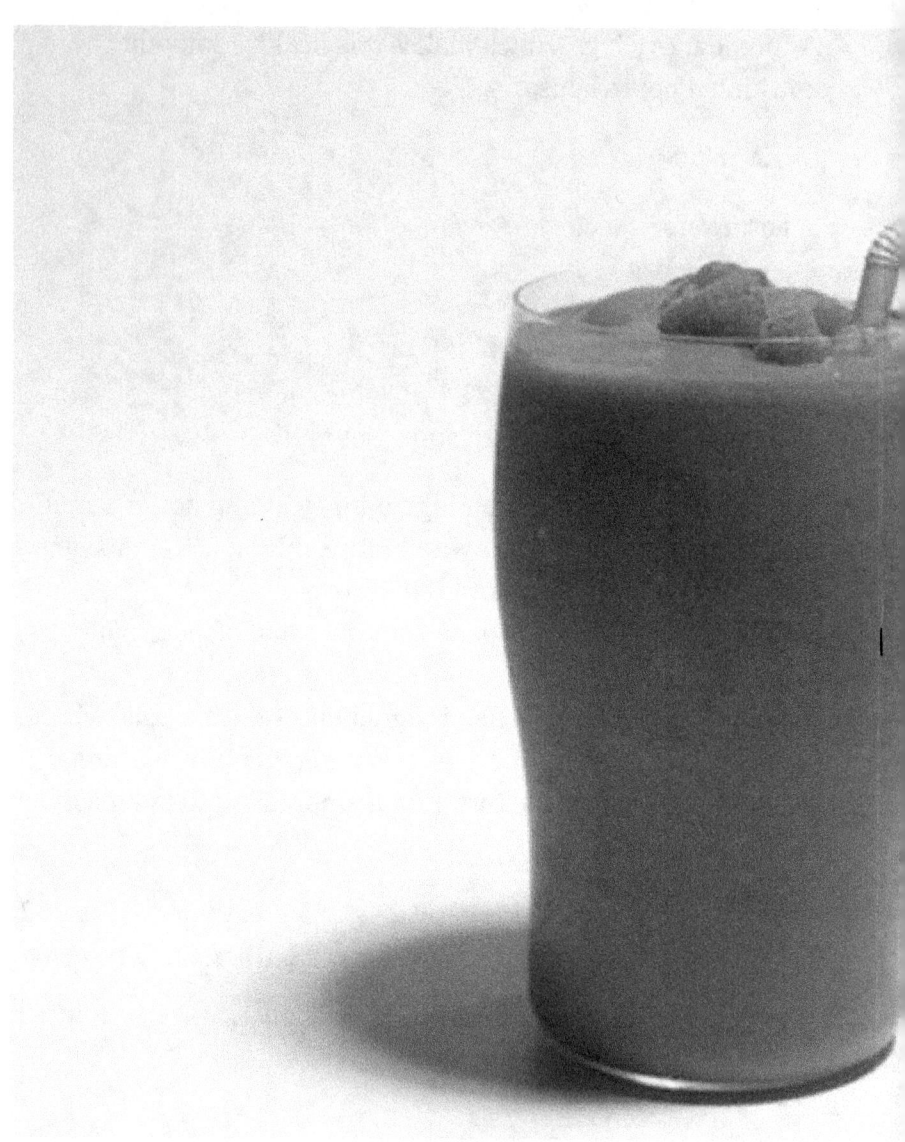

Very Berry Breakfast

Start your day off with a bang with this fruit-packed smoothie recipe.

SERVINGS: 2

1 c frozen unsweetened raspberries
¾ c chilled unsweetened almond or rice milk

¼ c frozen pitted unsweetened cherries or raspberries
1½ Tbsp honey
2 tsp finely grated fresh ginger
1 tsp ground flaxseed
2 tsp fresh lemon juice

COMBINE all ingredients in blender, adding lemon juice to taste. Puree until smooth. Pour into 2 chilled glasses.

NUTRITION (per serving) 112 cals, 1.5 g fat, 0 g sat fat, 56 mg sodium, 25.5 g carbs, 20 g sugars, 3 g fiber, 1 g protein

MORE: 12 Healthy Breakfasts For All-Day Energy

5/21

World's Best Smoothie

World's Best Smoothie

Slurp down this smoothie recipe at breakfast, and you'll feel satisfied until lunchtime.

SERVINGS: 1

1 c plain nonfat yogurt
1 banana
½ c orange juice
6 frozen strawberries

COMBINE the yogurt, banana, juice, and strawberries for 20 seconds. Scrape down the sides and blend for an additional 15 seconds.

NUTRITION (per serving) 300 cal, 14 g pro, 63 g carb, 5 g fiber, 45 g sugars, 0.5 g fat, 0 g sat fat, 180 mg sodium

MORE: 20 Superb Strawberry Recipes

Pineapple Passion

Pineapple Passion

This decadently thick smoothie recipe can even satisfy your desire for ice cream and it's healthy!

SERVINGS: 1

1 c low-fat or light vanilla yogurt
6 ice cubes
1 c pineapple chunks

1. COMBINE the yogurt and ice cubes. Blend, pulsing as needed, until the ice is in large chunks.
2. ADD the pineapple and blend at "whip" speed until smooth.

NUTRITION (per serving) 283 cals, 3.5 g fat, 2 g sat fat, 167 mg sodium, 53.5 g carbs, 48 g sugars, 2 g fiber, 13 g protein

Strawberry-Kiwi Smoothie

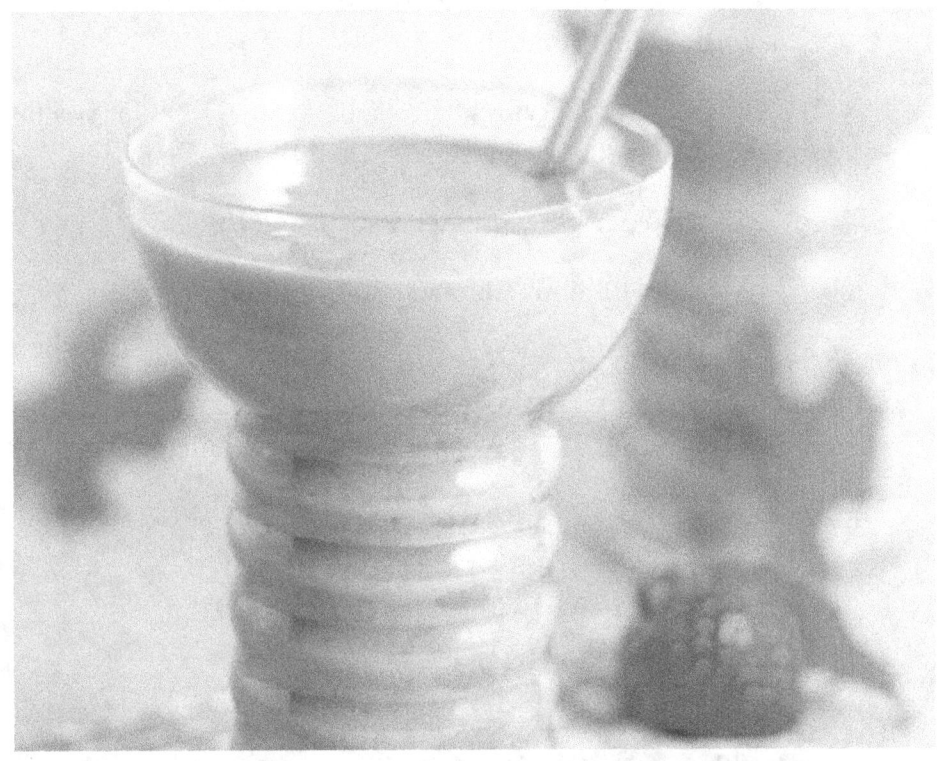

Strawberry-Kiwi Smoothie

Stay full and fight disease. This high-fiber smoothie recipe becomes even healthier when you use organic kiwis, which contain higher levels of heart-healthy polyphenols and vitamin C.

SERVINGS: 4

1¼ c cold apple juice
1 ripe banana, sliced
1 kiwifruit, sliced

5 frozen strawberries
1½ tsp honey

COMBINE the juice, banana, kiwifruit, strawberries, and honey. Blend until smooth.

NUTRITION (per serving) 87 cals, 0.3 g fat, 0 g sat fat, 3.5 mg sodium, 22 g carbs, 16.5 g sugars, 1.5 g fiber, 0.5 g protein

MORE: Sip Your Way Smarter With These Yummy Recipes

Banana-Blueberry-Soy Smoothie

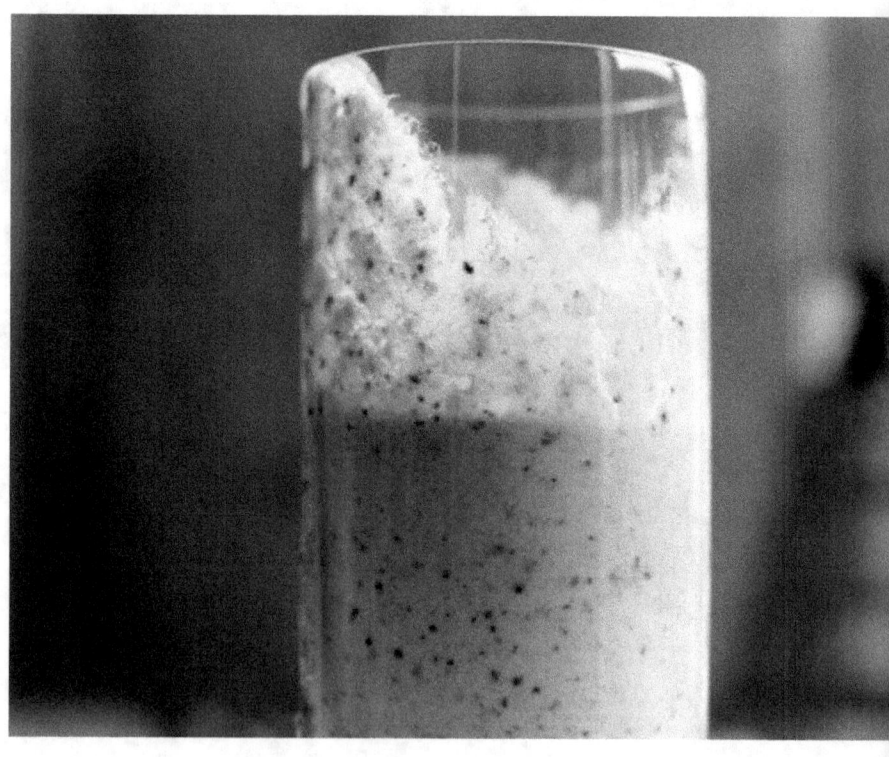

Banana-Blueberry-Soy Smoothie

Succulent, summer-ripe blueberries burst with flavor in this delicious smoothie. Skip the sugar or artificial sweetener for a healthier pick; the fruit makes it naturally sweet.

SERVINGS: 2

1¼ c light soy milk
½ c frozen loose-pack blueberries
½ frozen banana, sliced
2 tsp sugar or 2 packets artificial sweetener
1 tsp pure vanilla extract

COMBINE 1 cup of the milk, the blueberries, banana, sugar or sweetener, and vanilla extract. Blend for 20 to 30 seconds, or until smooth. Add up to ¼ cup more milk if a thinner smoothie is desired.

NUTRITION (per serving) 125 cals, 1.5 g fat, 0.1 g sat fat, 60 mg sodium, 25 g carbs, 11 g sugars, 2 g fiber, 3 g protein

MORE: 8 Blender Recipes Starring Peanut Butter

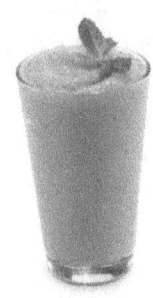

Tropical Papaya Perfection

Thick like a milkshake, this coconut-infused smoothie recipe transports you to a tropical island.

SERVINGS: 1

1 papaya, cut into chunks
1 c fat-free plain yogurt
½ c fresh pineapple chunks
½ c crushed ice
1 tsp coconut extract
1 tsp ground flaxseed

COMBINE the papaya, yogurt, pineapple, ice, coconut extract, and flaxseed. Process for about 30 seconds, or until smooth and frosty.

NUTRITION (per serving) 299 cals, 1.5 g fat, 0.1 g sat fat, 149 mg sodium, 64 g carbs, 44 g sugars, 7 g fiber, 13 g protein

MORE: 10 Foods That Lower Cholesterol

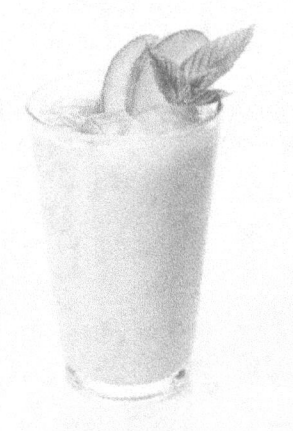

Just Peachy

Fat-free vanilla ice cream makes this protein packed smoothie sinful and slimming. Skip the spoonful of sugar for a healthier pick.

SERVINGS: 2

1 c 1% milk
2 Tbsp low-fat vanilla yogurt
½ c frozen peaches
½ c strawberries
⅛ tsp powdered ginger
2 tsp whey protein powder (such as Source Organic Whey Protein)
3 ice cubes

1. BLEND together any liquid ingredients (milk, yogurt, juice, etc.) and protein powder; this will help break down the grainy powder and make sure it's evenly distributed.
2. ADD mushy ingredients, like precooked oatmeal and fruit, then add ice at the end. For a thicker shake, you can toss in more ice cubes; you'll add volume without the calories.

NUTRITION (per serving) 150 cals, 2 g fat, 1 g sat fat, 73 mg sodium, 26.5 g carbs, 24 g sugars, 2 g fiber, 9 g protein

MORE: 10 Powder-Free Ways To Add Protein To Your Drink

Apricot-Mango Madness

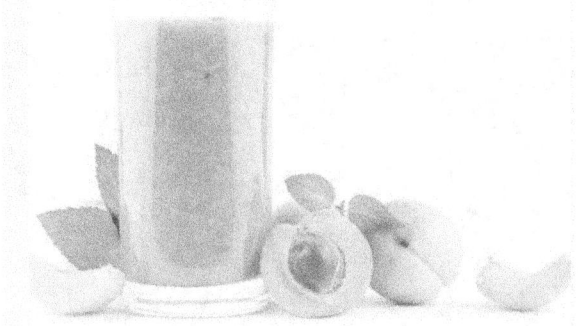

Apricot-Mango Madness

Fresh lemon juice adds a tangy splash to this sweet smoothie.

SERVINGS: 2

6 apricots, peeled, pitted, and chopped (about 2 c)
2 ripe mangoes, 10 to 12 ounces each, peeled and chopped (about 2 c)
1 c reduced-fat milk or plain low-fat yogurt
4 tsp fresh lemon juice
¼ tsp vanilla extract
8 ice cubes
Lemon peel twists (garnish)

1. PLACE the apricots, mangoes, milk or yogurt, lemon juice, and vanilla extract in a blender. Process for 8 seconds. Add the ice cubes, and process 6 to 8 seconds longer, or until smooth.
2. POUR into tall glasses, garnish with lemon twists, if desired, and serve immediately.

NUTRITION (per serving) 252 cals, 3.5 g fat, 1.5 g sat fat, 57 mg sodium, 53 g carbs, 45.5 g sugars, 6 g fiber, 7 g protein

MORE: Lose The Bloat With These 25 Slimming Sassy Water Recipes

Watermelon Wonder

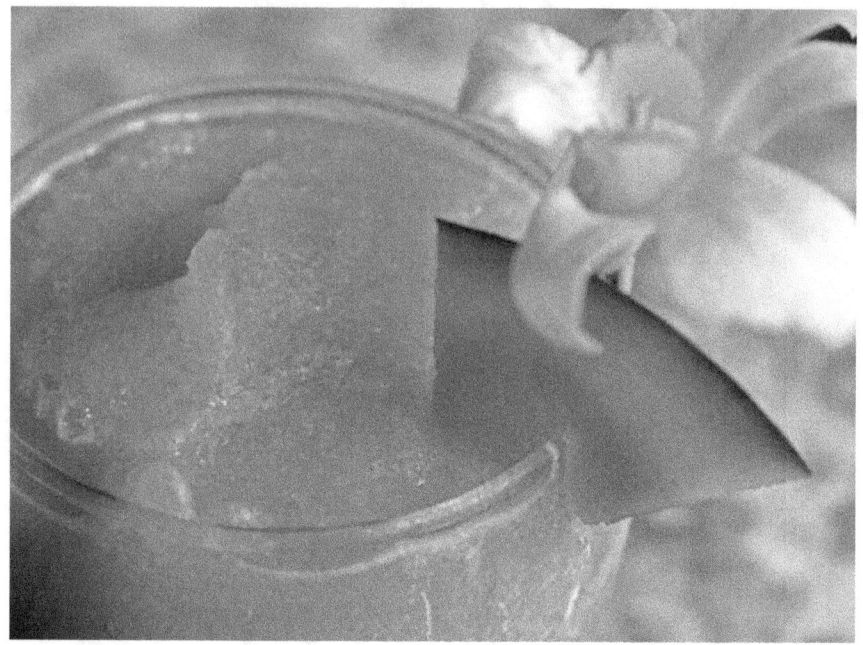

Watermelon Wonder

Transform a summer fruit favorite into a delightful healthy smoothie. Just remember to buy seedless watermelon or remove the seeds before you blend!

SERVINGS: 2

2 c chopped watermelon
¼ c fat-free milk
2 c ice

COMBINE the watermelon and milk, and blend for 15 seconds, or until smooth. Add the ice, and blend 20 seconds longer, or to your desired consistency. Add more ice, if needed, and blend for 10 seconds.

NUTRITION (per serving) 56 cals, 0.3 g fat, 0 g sat fat, 19.5 mg sodium, 13 g carbs, 11 g sugars, 0.5 g fiber, 2 g protein

MORE: This Is Your Body On Diet Soda (Infographic)

Berry Good Workout Smoothie

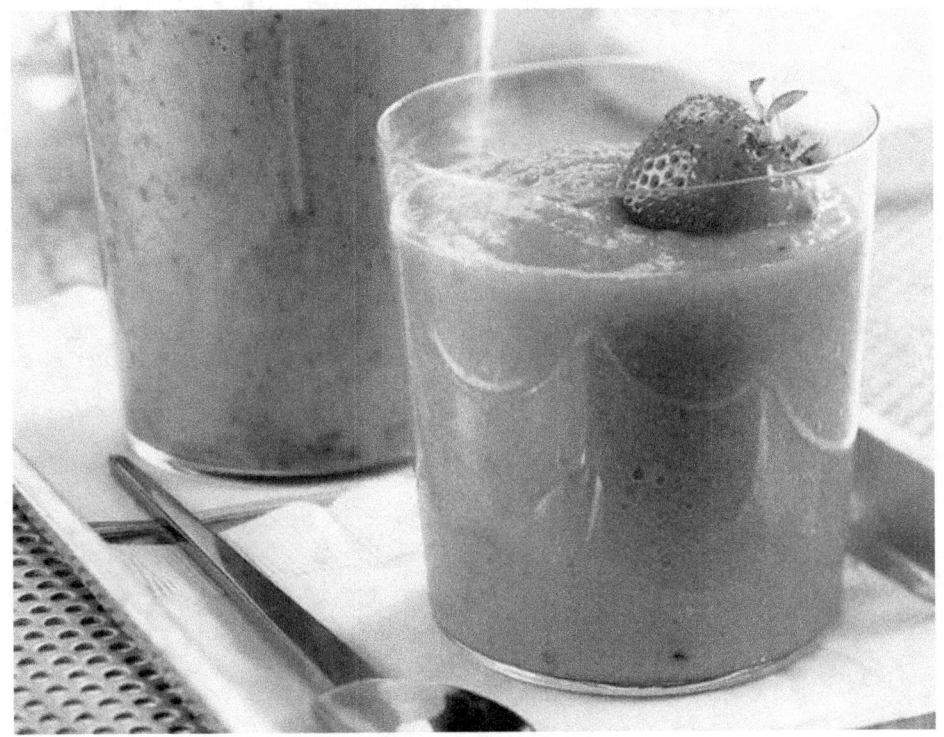

Berry Good Workout Smoothie

Get the energy you need to power through your workout in minutes with this easy-to-make smoothie recipe. For an extra dose of calcium, try adding a teaspoon of Organic Kale Powder.

SERVINGS: 1

1½ c chopped strawberries
1 c blueberries
½ c raspberries
2 Tbsp honey

1 tsp fresh lemon juice
½ c ice cubes

BLEND all ingredients.

NUTRITION (per serving) 162.5 cals, 1 g fat, 0.1 g sat fat, 5 mg sodium, 41.5 g carbs, 32 g sugars, 6 g fiber, 2 g protein

MORE: 7 Ways To Boost Your Energy Without Caffeine

14/21

Sunrise Smoothie

MOTIVATIONAL QUOTES

1. **Remember! No Pain, No Gain.**

2. **Stay mentally, physically, emotionally, financially and spiritually fit.**

3. **Be safe and build, be safe and build.**

4. **Let's go! Get in "Beast mode" my friends.**

5. **Hard work, Dedication – Rest your muscles every other day.**

6. For the serious lifters and future Mr. and Ms. Olympians and Olympia's. "Live, Love and Lift."

7. Whether it's the tough, grunting "Terror Dome" part of the gym or the "No-Judgment" zone, Go in!!!

8. Your body is your temple, threat it as such. Mind, Body and Soul, (May the Lord Bless your Body.)

9. Time to put work in. Make the donuts so we can "Eat" and cash some checks at the Buff Bank (It's a gym work out thing you have to understand.)

10. Don't let your upper body get too far ahead of your body. Spend time on your legs.

11. Rest when you have to (Your muscles, mind and total body) but never ever quit on yourself, our health depends on it.

12. A half hour workout is only 2% of your day, no excuses.

13. You can feel sure tomorrow or you can feel sorry tomorrow. You choose.

14. Suck it up now so you don't have to suck it up later.

15. Train like a beast to look like a beauty.

16. Today is your day to start fresh and to eat right to train hard, to live healthy, and to be proud (Bonnie Pfiester)

17. The only bad workout is the one that didn't happen. "Showing up is half the workout."

18. Don't be afraid of a little sweat. "Fat is just fat crying."

19. When you feel like quitting think about why you started.

20. You're only one workout away from a good mood.

21. Just one more, "You Got This."

22. It's all About the Body, Mind and Soul.

Fitness Jokes

1. The trouble with jogging is that, by the time you realize you're not in shape for it, it's too far to walk back. – (Franklin P. Jones)

2. Whenever I feel like exercising, I lie down until the feeling passes. (Robert M. Hutchins)

3. Doctor to patient: "What fits your busy schedule better, exercising one hour a day or being dead 24 hours a day? (Randy Glasbergen)

4. The word "aerobics" came about when the gym instructors got together and said: If we're going to charge $ an hour we can't call it "Jumping up and down" (Rita Rudner)

5. Husband to wife: "My doctor told me to start my exercise program very gradually. Today I drove by a store that sells sweatpants." (Randy Glasbergen)

6. I'd be more of a fan of exercising if calories screamed when you burned them. (Jehmeh)

7. I prefer sit-ups to jumping jacks. At least I get to lie down after each one.

8. A man asked a trainer in the gym: "I want to impress that beautiful girl, which machine can I use? The trainer replied; use the ATM machine outside the gym.

9. I have flabby thighs, but fortunately my stomach covers them.

10. I joined a health club for $400 a year and haven't lost a pound. Apparently you have to show up?

Top 20 Gyms in America to Date

- Planet Fitness   - X Sport
  Fitness
- Blink   - Crunch
- Equinox   - UFC
- L.A. Fitness   - YMCA
- Metro Flex   - Golds
  Gym
- Crossfit Hardcore   - Lifetime
  Fitness
- Anytime Fitness   - Crunch
  Fit
- NY Health & Racquet Club   - The
  Sport Club
- 24hr Fitness   - Eclipse

*Some Interesting and Effective Foods to be A Healthier Human-Being

1. Almonds
2. Apricots
3. Bananas
4. Beets
5. Berries (Frozen)
6. Cayenne
7. Chia Seeds
8. Cinnamon
9. Citrus fruit
10. Coconut
11. Apricots
12. Flax seeds
13. Grapes
14. Green tea powder
15. Ginger
16. Oats
17. Plant-based protein powder
18. Pomegranate
19. Spinach
20. Tofu

The Best Healthiest Diets

1. **Flexitarian** – Emphasizes fruit, veggies, plant based protein. Basically mean be a vegetarian most of the time and indulge in meat occasionally. (A flexible diet)

2. **Mind Diet** – Prevents Alzheimer disease with brain healthy foods, blends tow healthy diets, the dash diet and the Mediterranean diet.

3. **Dash Diet** – Dietary approaches to stop hypertension, developed to fight high blood pressure. Potassium, calcium, protein and fiber are crucial to fending off high blood pressure.

4. **Volumetrics** – An eating guideline. Food is divided into four categories. Very low density, medium density and high density. Far more info "research "Volumetric."

5. **Mayo Clinic** – Claims you can lose up to 6-10 pounds in 2 weeks with a healthy diet program based on a diet created by The Mayo Clinic.

6. **Weight Watchers** – An open and complex diet. For more details and in depth information Google and research (Weight Watchers Diet)

7. **Fertility**- Encourages healthy pregnancy and helps you get pregnant. Boost ovulation and improve fertility (Research details).

8. **<u>Jenny Craig</u>**- Pre-packed meals restricting calories, fat and portions.

9. **<u>Mediterranean Diet</u>** – Vegetables, Whole grains, legumes, fruits, nuts, olive oil tasty, herbs and spices. Moderate wine drinking encouraged. A heart healthy diet.

10. **<u>TLC</u>** – (Therapeutic Lifestyle Changes) A low fat way of eating that involves munching on fruit, veggie, whole grains, fish and skin free poultry.

Some of The Best Weight Loss Diets

1. **Vegan**- Don't eat any animal products, while vegetarians eliminate meat, fish and poultry, vegans also exclude dairy and eggs but eat greens, fruit , grains, nuts.

2. **Biggest Loser** – consist of eating plenty of fruits and vegetables, having a food journal, minimal red meat and regular exercise and can prevent some major illnesses.

3. **Atkins** – Fatty foods gone, no sweets and bread. Protein and fat-like chicken, meat and eggs are embraced.

4. **South Beach** – A high fiber, low-glycemic carbohydrates, unsaturated fats and lean protein diet.

5. **Raw Food** – Packed with natural enzymes and nutrients that help the body reach optimal health. Fruits and vegetable dominate this diet.

6. **Slim Fast** – Shakes, meal bars and snack bars replace breakfast, lunch and snacks restricting calories and portion sizes. Have a 500 calorie meal each day for balance.

7. **HMR Program** – (Health Management Resources) Meal replacements, low calorie shakes, multigrain to cereal, fruits and vegetables.

8. **<u>Spark Solution</u>** – A detailed guide of meal plans and exercise routines for 2 weeks. The Spark Solution book provides follow-up guidance.

9. **<u>Engine 2</u>** – Eliminating "Junk" such as meat, dairy, refined and processed foods and fully embracing tasty, nutritious, whole plant based foods.

10. **<u>Weight Watchers</u>** – An open and complex diet. Far more details and in-depth information Google (Weight Watchers Diet)

Also: Dash, Mayo, Volumetrics, Flexitarian, Weight Watchers and Jenny Craig diets which are also on the list of best healthiest diets. Try organic foods also.

THIRTY DAY CHALLENGES

30 DAY ARMS CHALLENGE

www.30dayfitnesschallenges.com

DAY 1	6 TRICEP DIPS / 4 PUSH UPS 8 MOUNTAIN CLIMBERS	DAY 16	8 TRICEP DIPS / 9 PUSH UPS 15 MOUNTAIN CLIMBERS
DAY 2	6 TRICEP DIPS / 4 PUSH UPS 8 MOUNTAIN CLIMBERS	DAY 17	10 TRICEP DIPS / 9 PUSH UPS 15 MOUNTAIN CLIMBERS
DAY 3	6 TRICEP DIPS / 5 PUSH UPS 10 MOUNTAIN CLIMBERS	DAY 18	10 TRICEP DIPS / 9 PUSH UPS 15 MOUNTAIN CLIMBERS
DAY 4	6 TRICEP DIPS / 5 PUSH UPS 10 MOUNTAIN CLIMBERS	DAY 19	REST DAY
DAY 5	REST DAY	DAY 20	10 TRICEP DIPS / 9 PUSH UPS 18 MOUNTAIN CLIMBERS
DAY 6	8 TRICEP DIPS / 6 PUSH UPS 10 MOUNTAIN CLIMBERS	DAY 21	10 TRICEP DIPS / 10 PUSH UPS 18 MOUNTAIN CLIMBERS
DAY 7	8 TRICEP DIPS / 6 PUSH UPS 12 MOUNTAIN CLIMBERS	DAY 22	10 TRICEP DIPS / 10 PUSH UPS 18 MOUNTAIN CLIMBERS
DAY 8	8 TRICEP DIPS / 8 PUSH UPS 12 MOUNTAIN CLIMBERS	DAY 23	10 TRICEP DIPS / 10 PUSH UPS 20 MOUNTAIN CLIMBERS
DAY 9	8 TRICEP DIPS / 8 PUSH UPS 15 MOUNTAIN CLIMBERS	DAY 24	10 TRICEP DIPS / 10 PUSH UPS 20 MOUNTAIN CLIMBERS
DAY 10	10 TRICEP DIPS / 8 PUSH UPS 15 MOUNTAIN CLIMBERS	DAY 25	10 TRICEP DIPS / 11 PUSH UPS 20 MOUNTAIN CLIMBERS
DAY 11	10 TRICEP DIPS / 8 PUSH UPS 15 MOUNTAIN CLIMBERS	DAY 26	REST DAY
DAY 12	REST DAY	DAY 27	12 TRICEP DIPS / 11 PUSH UPS 22 MOUNTAIN CLIMBERS
DAY 13	8 TRICEP DIPS / 8 PUSH UPS 12 MOUNTAIN CLIMBERS	DAY 28	12 TRICEP DIPS / 11 PUSH UPS 22 MOUNTAIN CLIMBERS
DAY 14	8 TRICEP DIPS / 8 PUSH UPS 12 MOUNTAIN CLIMBERS	DAY 29	12 TRICEP DIPS / 11 PUSH UPS 22 MOUNTAIN CLIMBERS
DAY 15	8 TRICEP DIPS / 9 PUSH UPS 12 MOUNTAIN CLIMBERS	DAY 30	12 TRICEP DIPS / 12 PUSH UPS 25 MOUNTAIN CLIMBERS

#30dayfitness   www.30dayfitnesschallenges.com   #30dayfitness

30 DAY TRICEP DIPS
CHALLENGE

www.30dayfitnesschallenges.com

DAY 1	5 TRICEP DIPS		DAY 16	50 TRICEP DIPS
DAY 2	10 TRICEP DIPS		DAY 17	55 TRICEP DIPS
DAY 3	15 TRICEP DIPS		DAY 18	60 TRICEP DIPS
DAY 4	20 TRICEP DIPS		DAY 19	65 TRICEP DIPS
DAY 5	REST DAY		DAY 20	REST DAY
DAY 6	20 TRICEP DIPS		DAY 21	65 TRICEP DIPS
DAY 7	25 TRICEP DIPS		DAY 22	70 TRICEP DIPS
DAY 8	30 TRICEP DIPS		DAY 23	75 TRICEP DIPS
DAY 9	35 TRICEP DIPS		DAY 24	80 TRICEP DIPS
DAY 10	REST DAY		DAY 25	REST DAY
DAY 11	35 TRICEP DIPS		DAY 26	80 TRICEP DIPS
DAY 12	40 TRICEP DIPS		DAY 27	85 TRICEP DIPS
DAY 13	45 TRICEP DIPS		DAY 28	90 TRICEP DIPS
DAY 14	50 TRICEP DIPS		DAY 29	95 TRICEP DIPS
DAY 15	REST DAY		DAY 30	100 TRICEP DIPS

#30dayfitness   www.30dayfitnesschallenges.com   #30dayfitness

30 DAY BURPEE CHALLENGE

www.30dayfitnesschallenges.com

DAY 1	5 BURPEES		DAY 16	50 BURPEES
DAY 2	10 BURPEES		DAY 17	55 BURPEES
DAY 3	15 BURPEES		DAY 18	60 BURPEES
DAY 4	20 BURPEES		DAY 19	65 BURPEES
DAY 5	REST DAY		DAY 20	REST DAY
DAY 6	20 BURPEES		DAY 21	65 BURPEES
DAY 7	25 BURPEES		DAY 22	70 BURPEES
DAY 8	30 BURPEES		DAY 23	75 BURPEES
DAY 9	35 BURPEES		DAY 24	80 BURPEES
DAY 10	REST DAY		DAY 25	REST DAY
DAY 11	35 BURPEES		DAY 26	80 BURPEES
DAY 12	40 BURPEES		DAY 27	85 BURPEES
DAY 13	45 BURPEES		DAY 28	90 BURPEES
DAY 14	50 BURPEES		DAY 29	95 BURPEES
DAY 15	REST DAY		DAY 30	100 BURPEES

 #30dayfitness   www.30dayfitnesschallenges.com   #30dayfitness

30 DAY EASY PUSH UP
CHALLENGE

www.30dayfitnesschallenges.com

DAY 1	3 PUSH UPS	DAY 16	REST DAY
DAY 2	4 PUSH UPS	DAY 17	12 PUSH UPS
DAY 3	5 PUSH UPS	DAY 18	14 PUSH UPS
DAY 4	REST DAY	DAY 19	15 PUSH UPS
DAY 5	5 PUSH UPS	DAY 20	REST DAY
DAY 6	6 PUSH UPS	DAY 21	15 PUSH UPS
DAY 7	7 PUSH UPS	DAY 22	16 PUSH UPS
DAY 8	REST DAY	DAY 23	17 PUSH UPS
DAY 9	7 PUSH UPS	DAY 24	REST DAY
DAY 10	8 PUSH UPS	DAY 25	17 PUSH UPS
DAY 11	9 PUSH UPS	DAY 26	18 PUSH UPS
DAY 12	REST DAY	DAY 27	19 PUSH UPS
DAY 13	9 PUSH UPS	DAY 28	REST DAY
DAY 14	11 PUSH UPS	DAY 29	19 PUSH UPS
DAY 15	12 PUSH UPS	DAY 30	20 PUSH UPS

 #30dayfitness   www.30dayfitnesschallenges.com   #30dayfitness

30-DAY FULL-BODY FITNESS CHALLENGE

Work your upper body, lower body and everything in between!

MONDAY + THURSDAY

100 Push-Ups

TUESDAY + FRIDAY

100 Squats

WEDNESDAY + SATURDAY

100 Crunches

SUNDAY

Rest, Repeat, or Test

BE SMART. BE SAFE. GET FIT. HAVE FUN!

www.FaceBook.com/30DayChallengeSeries
www.eatdrinkandbeskinny.com

30 DAY LUNGE CHALLENGE

www.30dayfitnesschallenges.com

DAY 1	20 LUNGES		DAY 16	REST DAY
DAY 2	25 LUNGES		DAY 17	90 LUNGES
DAY 3	30 LUNGES		DAY 18	95 LUNGES
DAY 4	35 LUNGES		DAY 19	100 LUNGES
DAY 5	40 LUNGES		DAY 20	105 LUNGES
DAY 6	45 LUNGES		DAY 21	110 LUNGES
DAY 7	50 LUNGES		DAY 22	115 LUNGES
DAY 8	REST DAY		DAY 23	120 LUNGES
DAY 9	55 LUNGES		DAY 24	REST DAY
DAY 10	60 LUNGES		DAY 25	125 LUNGES
DAY 11	65 LUNGES		DAY 26	130 LUNGES
DAY 12	70 LUNGES		DAY 27	135 LUNGES
DAY 13	75 LUNGES		DAY 28	140 LUNGES
DAY 14	80 LUNGES		DAY 29	145 LUNGES
DAY 15	85 LUNGES		DAY 30	150 LUNGES

#30dayfitness   www.30dayfitnesschallenges.com   #30dayfitness

30 DAY PLANK CHALLENGE

www.30dayfitnesschallenges.com

DAY 1	20 SECONDS		DAY 16	120 SECONDS
DAY 2	20 SECONDS		DAY 17	120 SECONDS
DAY 3	30 SECONDS		DAY 18	150 SECONDS
DAY 4	30 SECONDS		DAY 19	REST DAY
DAY 5	40 SECONDS		DAY 20	150 SECONDS
DAY 6	REST DAY		DAY 21	150 SECONDS
DAY 7	45 SECONDS		DAY 22	180 SECONDS
DAY 8	45 SECONDS		DAY 23	180 SECONDS
DAY 9	60 SECONDS		DAY 24	210 SECONDS
DAY 10	60 SECONDS		DAY 25	210 SECONDS
DAY 11	60 SECONDS		DAY 26	REST DAY
DAY 12	90 SECONDS		DAY 27	240 SECONDS
DAY 13	REST DAY		DAY 28	240 SECONDS
DAY 14	90 SECONDS		DAY 29	270 SECONDS
DAY 15	90 SECONDS		DAY 30	300 SECONDS

#30dayfitness   www.30dayfitnesschallenges.com   #30dayfitness

30 DAY BUTT CHALLENGE

www.30dayfitnesschallenges.com

DAY 1	15 SQUATS / 5 BRIDGES 10 LUNGES		**DAY 16**	55 SQUATS / 35 BRIDGES 40 LUNGES
DAY 2	20 SQUATS / 5 BRIDGES 10 LUNGES		**DAY 17**	55 SQUATS / 35 BRIDGES 40 LUNGES
DAY 3	20 SQUATS / 10 BRIDGES 15 LUNGES		**DAY 18**	55 SQUATS / 40 BRIDGES 45 LUNGES
DAY 4	25 SQUATS / 10 BRIDGES 15 LUNGES		**DAY 19**	60 SQUATS / 40 BRIDGES 45 LUNGES
DAY 5	30 SQUATS / 10 BRIDGES 20 LUNGES		**DAY 20**	60 SQUATS / 40 BRIDGES 50 LUNGES
DAY 6	30 SQUATS / 15 BRIDGES 20 LUNGES		**DAY 21**	65 SQUATS / 45 BRIDGES 50 LUNGES
DAY 7	35 SQUATS / 15 BRIDGES 20 LUNGES		**DAY 22**	65 SQUATS / 45 BRIDGES 50 LUNGES
DAY 8	35 SQUATS / 20 BRIDGES 25 LUNGES		**DAY 23**	65 SQUATS / 50 BRIDGES 55 LUNGES
DAY 9	35 SQUATS / 20 BRIDGES 25 LUNGES		**DAY 24**	70 SQUATS / 50 BRIDGES 55 LUNGES
DAY 10	40 SQUATS / 20 BRIDGES 30 LUNGES		**DAY 25**	70 SQUATS / 50 BRIDGES 60 LUNGES
DAY 11	40 SQUATS / 25 BRIDGES 30 LUNGES		**DAY 26**	70 SQUATS / 55 BRIDGES 50 LUNGES
DAY 12	45 SQUATS / 25 BRIDGES 30 LUNGES		**DAY 27**	75 SQUATS / 55 BRIDGES 65 LUNGES
DAY 13	45 SQUATS / 30 BRIDGES 35 LUNGES		**DAY 28**	75 SQUATS / 60 BRIDGES 65 LUNGES
DAY 14	50 SQUATS / 30 BRIDGES 35 LUNGES		**DAY 29**	80 SQUATS / 60 BRIDGES 70 LUNGES
DAY 15	50 SQUATS / 30 BRIDGES 40 LUNGES		**DAY 30**	90 SQUATS / 60 BRIDGES 70 LUNGES

#30dayfitness   www.30dayfitnesschallenges.com   #30dayfitness

Disclaimer: I am not a certified trainer, nutritionist or any professional along the lines of a fitness or health expert. The content in this book comes strictly from my opinion. Please seek advice from the proper health and fitness professional before taking any supplemental drugs or doing any kind of exercise.

E.Z. BLACKMAN

Also available in the "My 100 Favorite Word" Franchise

- Hip-hop Lyrics -

- Happy & Healthy - Money - Bible

-Entrepreneur -

COMING SOON

Under "My 100 Favorite Word" Franchise

- Law - College - Writers -
- Quotes -

E. Z. BLACKMAN

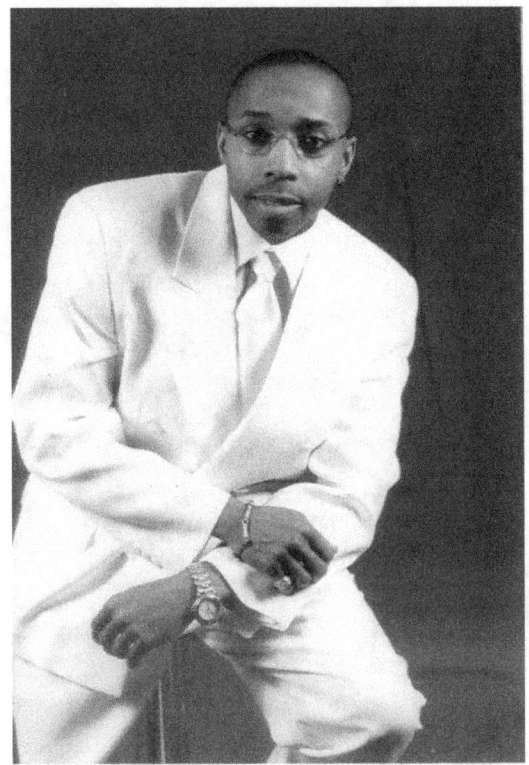

ABOUT THE AUTHOR

Edgar "EZ" Blackman, certified Chaplain, new author and aspiring motivational speaker from Brooklyn, N.Y. He loves to inspire and encourage anyone who wants and needs to be inspired and motivated. He is a member of the prestigious Toastmasters Int'l Organization, an avid Yogi, and an Army Veteran. He is one who never imagined of becoming an author or motivational speaker. Through faith, wisdom and a burning desire to find his purpose in life despite coming from humble beginnings and no particular goals in mind up until young adulthood.

Look for future uplifting books by EZ, and for speaking engagements or to host an event, contact EZ at: ezevthing@yahoo.com, on Facebook - EZ Blackman, Instagram: EZEVERYTHING, and on Twitter: EZ BLACKMAN.

Other books by E.Z. Blackman

 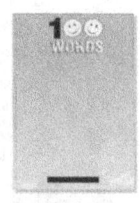 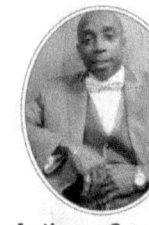 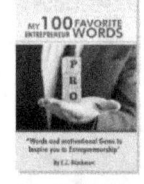 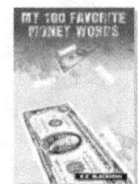

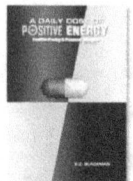 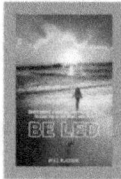 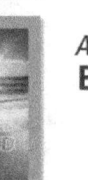 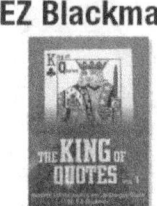 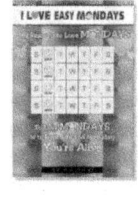 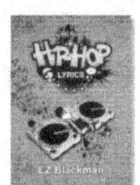

www.ingramcontent.com/pod-product-compliance
Lightning Source LLC
Chambersburg PA
CBHW060154290526
45789CB00003B/1036